IUI: Intrauterine Insemination

All you need to know

Dr. Sheila Harrison

Disclaimer

This content is not a substitute for consulting a professional physician but to give a fair knowledge about the disease and to equip you to seek medical assistance as early as possible if need be to avoid complications. It should also be noted that the area of medical science is a constantly changing field and due to the ever developing and changing nature of medical knowledge, we suggest you seek expert advice if you spot any discrepancies or decide to take action in reaction to the information in this content. Never reject medical advice from professionals or put off getting treatment because of something you read online, acquired through this material, or any other online resource.

And remember the internet won't heal you but God through Physicians will.

Table of Content

Introduction

IUI (Intrauterine Insemination) is a fertility treatment that offers hope to couples struggling to conceive. It involves the direct placement of prepared sperm into a woman's uterus during her fertile period. This increases the likelihood of successful fertilization and pregnancy. This article provides an in-depth look at Intrauterine Insemination (IUI), exploring it in detail.

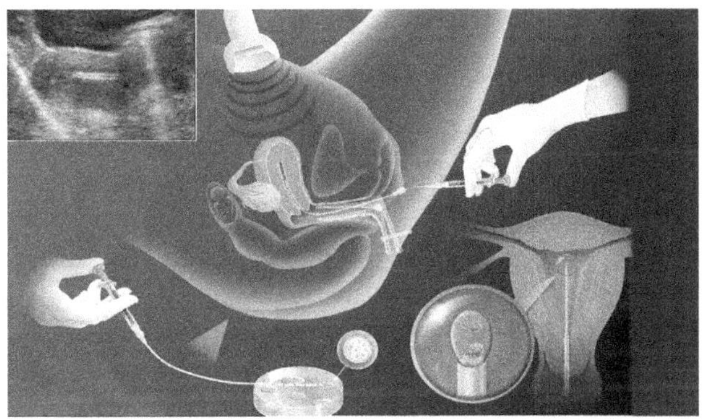

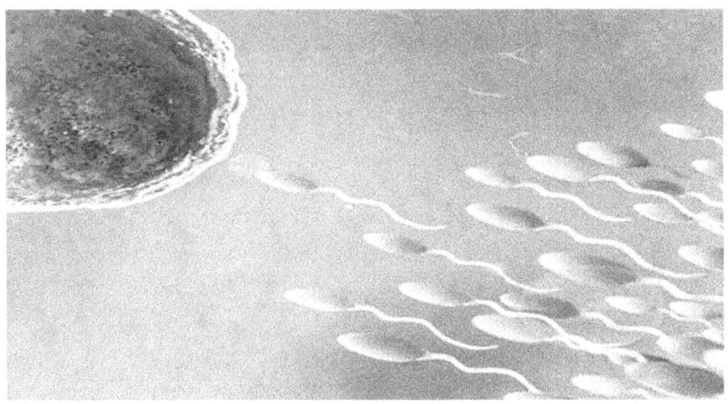

Section 1

What is IUI?

Intrauterine insemination (IUI), a type of artificial insemination for a fertility treatment where sperm is placed directly into a person's uterus. In this procedure, the doctors introduce concentrated and motile sperm into a woman's uterus to facilitate fertilization. The goal of Intrauterine Insemination(IUI) is to increase the number of sperm that reach the fallopian tubes, enhancing the likelihood of sperm meeting the egg and achieving pregnancy.

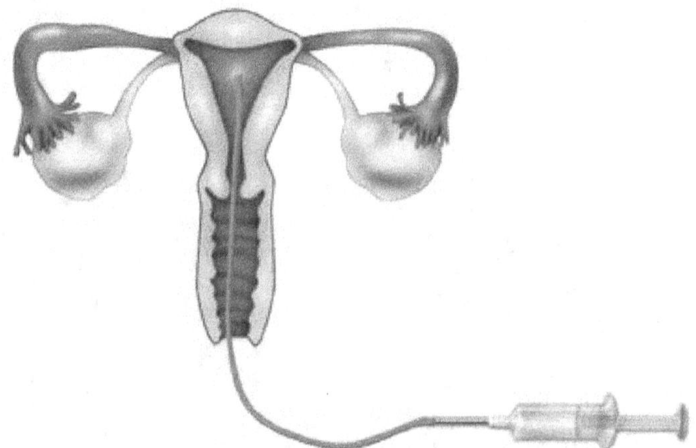

During a natural conception, sperm has to travel from your vagina through your cervix, into your uterus and to your fallopian tubes. Only 5% of the sperm are able to travel from your vagina to your uterus. Once your ovary releases an egg, it travels to your fallopian tube. This is where the sperm and egg meet and fertilization occurs. With IUI, the sperm is collected, washed and concentrated so that only high-quality sperm remain. This sperm is placed directly into your uterus with a catheter (thin tube), putting it closer to your fallopian tubes. IUI makes it easier for the sperm to reach an egg because it cuts down on the time and distance it has to travel. This increases your chance of becoming pregnant.

Healthcare providers often try IUI before other more invasive and expensive fertility treatments. IUIs can be performed with your partner's sperm or with donor sperm. A person may take fertility drugs to ensure eggs are released during ovulation.

How and why did IUI come to be as a fertility treatment option?

The concept of artificial insemination dates back to ancient times. However, significant progress was made in the early 20th century, developing IUI as a fertility treatment option. In the 1940s, pioneers like Dr Gregory Pincus and Dr John Rock conducted groundbreaking research on reproductive biology and hormonal treatments, paving the way for modern fertility treatments like IUI.

People choose IUI for many reasons, such as infertility issues, or as a reproductive option for same-sex female couples or females who wish to have a baby without a partner, using a sperm donor.

Intrauterine insemination (IUI) may be used when these conditions are present:

- **Cervical mucus problems or other problems with your cervix:** Your cervix separates your vagina and uterus from each other. Mucus produced by your cervix helps sperm travel from your vagina, through your uterus and to your fallopian tubes. Thick mucus can make it hard for sperm to swim. With IUI, sperm bypasses your cervix and goes directly to your uterus.

- **Low sperm count or other sperm impairments:** Semen analysis is part of infertility treatment. It may show that your partner's sperm is small, weak, slow or oddly shaped, or that your partner doesn't have much sperm. IUI can help these problems because only high-quality sperm is selected and used in your treatment.

- **You're using donor sperm:** IUI is used when people use sperm from a person who isn't the birth parent's partner. This is called donor insemination (DI). DI is done when one partner has no sperm or when the sperm quality is so low that the sperm can't be used. Single women or same-sex female couples who wish to conceive can also use donor sperm.

- **Ejaculation or erection dysfunction:** IUI can be used when one partner can't get or sustain an erection or isn't able to ejaculate.

- **Semen allergy:** In rare cases, people have an allergy to their partner's semen. It can cause burning, swelling and redness in their vagina. IUI can be effective because the proteins causing the allergy are removed during sperm washing.

- **Unexplained infertility:** This is when healthcare providers can't find the cause for infertility.

Ideal candidates for IUI

IUI is a suitable fertility treatment for various groups of individuals and couples facing specific challenges in conceiving naturally. Ideal candidates for the procedure include:

- Couples with unexplained infertility: When all standard fertility evaluations yield no apparent cause for infertility, IUI may be a viable option.
- Mild male factor infertility: Couples facing male infertility due to low sperm count, decreased motility, or abnormal sperm shape may benefit from IUI.
- Cervical factor infertility: Women with cervical issues that hinder sperm passage

through the cervix may find success with IUI.

- Ovulation disorders: Women who experience irregular or absent ovulation can benefit from IUI when combined with ovulation-stimulating medications.
- Mild endometriosis: IUI can be an appropriate initial treatment for women with mild endometriosis.

The IUI process from beginning to end

The timeline for the IUI procedure is approximately four weeks (around 28 days) from beginning to end. It's about the same length as a regular menstrual cycle.

- Before starting the IUI process, you (and your partner) will have a thorough examination that could include bloodwork, semen analysis, ultrasound and other diagnostics.
- Some people are given oral fertility medicine for five days or injectable

medication for up to two weeks. This increases your chances of ovulation and releasing multiple eggs. Not all people require these medications.

- Insemination is a quick process. It takes a few minutes to insert the sperm. Your healthcare provider may ask you to lie down for around 15 minutes afterward.

- You can take a pregnancy test two weeks after insemination.

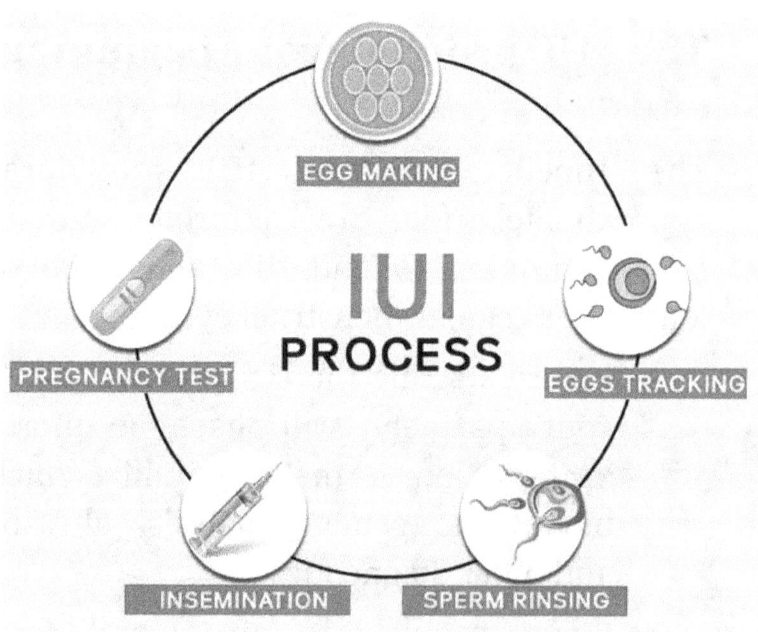

Section 2

The Preparation Process Before IUI Treatment

Before starting on an IUI cycle, certain preparatory steps are pivotal to optimize the chances of success. These preparations include:

- **Fertility Evaluation:** Both partners should undergo a thorough fertility evaluation to identify any underlying issues that may affect the IUI outcome. This evaluation involves assessing the woman's ovarian reserve, fallopian tube patency, and uterine health and conducting a semen analysis for the male partner.

- **Ovulation Prediction:** Accurate ovulation prediction is vital for the success of IUI. This may involve tracking the woman's menstrual cycle using several methods. These include basal body temperature charting, ovulation predictor kits, or monitoring hormonal changes.

- **Sexual Abstinence:** It is essential for the male partner to abstain from ejaculation for 2 to 3 days before the IUI procedure to ensure the highest concentration of sperm in the semen sample.

Lifestyle changes that may improve the success of IUI

Lifestyle factors play a significant role in fertility, and making certain adjustments can positively impact the success of IUI. Consider the following lifestyle changes:

- **Maintain a healthy diet:** A well-balanced diet rich in fruits, vegetables, whole grains, and lean proteins supports overall health and fertility. Antioxidant-rich foods, such as berries and nuts, may also boost reproductive health.

- **Exercise regularly:** Moderate and regular physical activity can enhance fertility and reduce stress. However, avoid excessive exercise, as it may negatively affect the IUI process.

- **Manage stress:** The state of anxiety affects the success of intrauterine insemination. Engaging in relaxation techniques such as yoga, meditation, or counseling may help manage stress.

- **Limit alcohol and caffeine intake:** Studies suggest a link between reduced fertility and excessive alcohol and caffeine consumption. Limiting these substances can benefit overall reproductive health.

- **Quit smoking:** Smoking has detrimental effects on fertility. Quitting smoking can improve the chances of successful IUI.

- **Maintain a healthy weight:** Both obesity and being underweight can impact fertility. Achieving and maintaining a healthy weight can optimize the chances of conception.

Clinical Examination / Test before IUI Treatment

Before starting IUI treatment, you'll need a thorough medical exam and fertility tests. Your partner will be examined and tested as well. This could include:

- A uterine exam.

- Ultrasounds of your uterus.

- A semen analysis.

- Screening for sexually transmitted infections (STIs) and other infectious diseases.

- Blood tests.

Your healthcare provider may recommend taking folic acid (included in most prenatal vitamins) at least three months before conception (or IUI treatment).

What to expect after IUI Treatment

There are some mild symptoms that you can experience after IUI:

- Mild cramping.

- Spotting for one or two days.

Most people will return to normal activities right away. You should avoid anything that makes you feel uncomfortable after IUI, but there usually aren't any restrictions. A pregnancy test can be taken around two weeks after IUI.

About Pain

Anesthesia isn't required for IUI and the procedure shouldn't be painful. However, you may have mild cramping and discomfort during and right after insemination.

IUI cost

The cost of IUI varies depending on the fertility clinic you use, your health history, use of medications and diagnostic testing. It's less expensive than other infertility treatments like IVF. You can expect to pay between $300 and $4,000 per cycle without insurance. Some states have laws that require insurance companies to cover part of the costs of infertility treatment.

Section 3

Medications used in IUI

IUI is often combined with fertility medications that stimulate your ovaries to produce and release as many eggs as possible. However, it's not always needed.

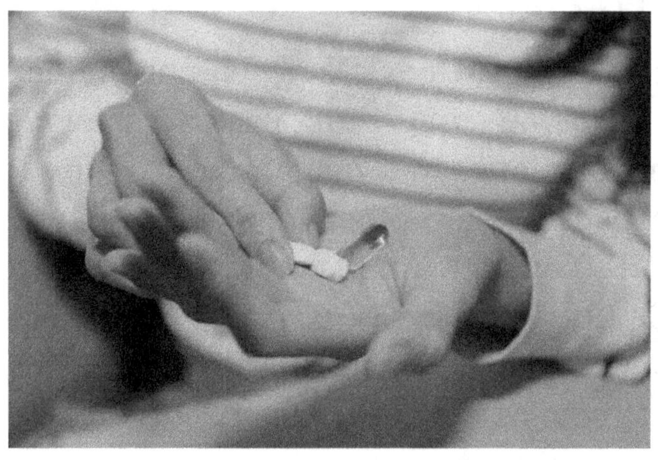

Types of medications

Doctors may prescribe several types of medications to induce ovulation to prepare the woman for IUI.

Some common medications are:

- **Clomiphene citrate (Clomid® or Serophene®):** This oral medication stimulates the release of hormones necessary for follicle development and ovulation.

- Letrozole (Femara®).

- **Gonadotropins:** Injectable hormones, such as follicle-stimulating hormone (FSH) and luteinizing hormone (LH), can be used to stimulate multiple follicles' growth.

- **Human Chorionic Gonadotropin (hCG):** An hCG injection is often administered when the follicles are mature, triggering ovulation and preparing for the procedure.

- Prenatal vitamins (recommended for all pregnancies).

Your healthcare provider will determine if fertility drugs will be used as part of your IUI treatment.

Administration

Clomiphene citrate is typically taken orally for a specific number of days in the menstrual cycle (5-9th in most cases), while gonadotropins are administered via subcutaneous injections.

Potential side effects

- Clomiphene citrate may cause hot flashes, gastrointestinal symptoms, breast discomfort, abnormal vaginal bleeding and headaches.

- Gonadotropins may lead to side effects such as local injection site reaction, gastrointestinal symptoms, such as nausea, abdominal pain, bloating, etc., and abdominal cramps, and may also cause OHSS in rare cases.

Section 4

Procedure Details

The IUI procedure involves several key steps. Firstly, the doctors monitor the woman's menstrual cycle carefully to determine the optimal time for insemination. If needed, they may prescribe fertility medications to stimulate the ovaries to produce multiple eggs, increasing the chances of successful conception. Below are the detailed steps.

The Detailed steps of IUI treatment

Every treatment plan and healthcare provider may have a slightly different process. IUI treatment typically includes the following:

Step 1: Ovulation

- Your healthcare provider will need to know exactly when you're ovulating. The timing of ovulation is critical to make sure sperm is injected at the right time.

- Determining the time of ovulation can be done using an at-home ovulation prediction kit that detects luteinizing hormone (LH). Your healthcare provider can also detect LH in blood tests. They may also use transvaginal ultrasound to look for signs of mature eggs. Sometimes, you're given an injection of human chorionic gonadotropin (hCG) or other fertility medications to make you ovulate one or more eggs. Ovulation typically occurs around 10 to 16 days after the first day of your period.

- Insemination (inserting the sperm into your uterus) usually occurs within 24 to 36 hours after LH is detected (either in your blood or urine), or after the hCG injection.

Step 2: Semen sample preparation

- Your partner provides a fresh sperm sample on the day of the IUI procedure. In some cases, your partner can provide the sample before and your healthcare provider can freeze it until it is time to be used. If you're using a sperm donor, the sample will be thawed and prepared.

- Sperm is prepared for insemination through a process called "sperm washing" that pulls out a concentrated amount of healthy sperm. If you're using donor sperm, the sperm bank usually sends sperm that's already washed.

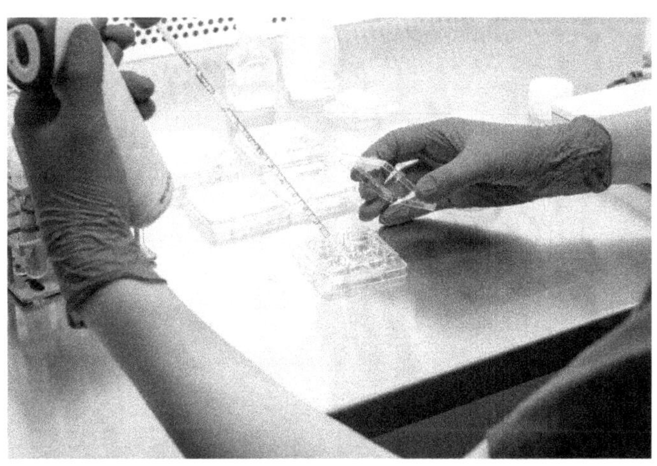

Step 3: Insemination

- The insemination procedure is simple and takes just a few minutes. You'll lie down on the exam table. Your healthcare provider will insert a speculum into your vagina — similar to what happens during a Pap test. Next, a catheter is inserted through your cervix into your uterus. Finally, your healthcare provider injects the washed sperm sample into your uterus.

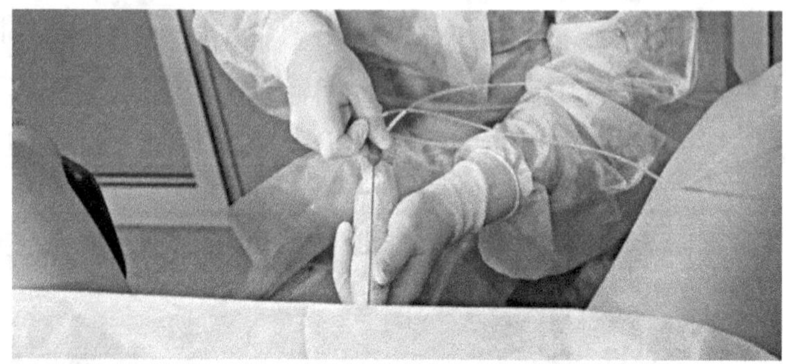

- You may be asked to lie down for 10 to 30 minutes after insemination. Pregnancy happens if sperm fertilizes an egg and the fertilized egg implants in the lining of your uterus.

- You may be given progesterone after IUI. Progesterone helps maintain the lining of your uterus and can improve the chances of implantation.

- You can take a pregnancy test approximately two weeks after IUI.

Please consult with your healthcare provider to get the best understanding of the IUI process and what to expect.

Step 4: Monitoring

Throughout the treatment cycle, the woman's progress is closely monitored through transvaginal ultrasounds and hormone level assessments. The size and number of mature follicles determined through transvaginal ultrasound help determine the timing of the insemination procedure.

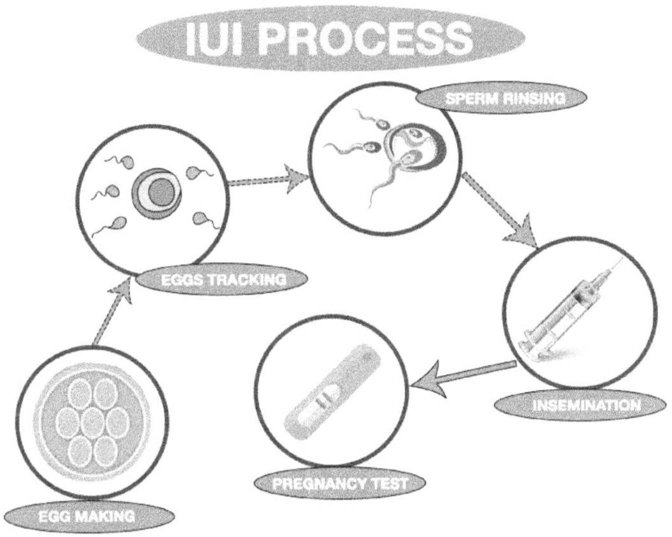

Section 5

Advantages and disadvantages of IUI compared to other fertility treatments

IUI significantly improves the chances of pregnancy by bypassing potential obstacles that sperm may encounter in their journey toward the egg. By placing the sperm directly into the uterus, the procedure enhances the concentration and proximity of sperm to the egg, optimizing the chances of fertilization. Additionally, the procedure's timing ensures that sperm is present in the fallopian tubes during ovulation when the egg is released, further increasing the likelihood of conception.

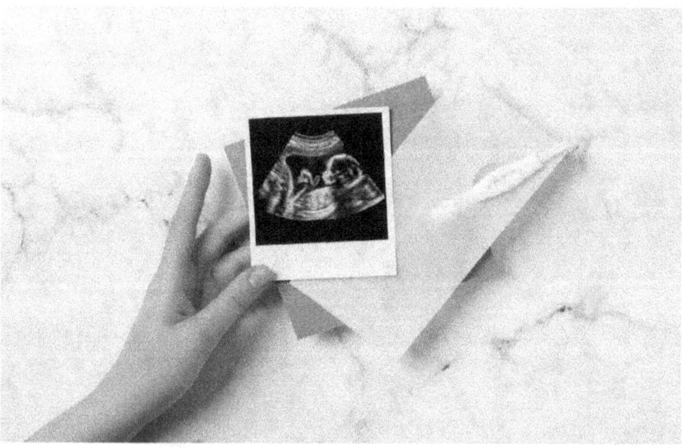

Advantages of IUI

- **Less invasive:** IUI is a minimally invasive procedure, involving no surgery or anesthesia.

- **Cost-effective:** Compared to more complex fertility treatments like IVF, IUI is generally more affordable.

- **Fewer side effects:** IUI has fewer side effects and a shorter recovery time than IVF.

- **Natural conception process:** IUI still relies on natural conception processes, making it a less drastic intervention.

- **Suitable for unexplained infertility:** IUI is a reasonable option when there is no identification of a specific cause of infertility.

Disadvantages of IUI

- Lower success rates: Compared to IVF, IUI has slightly lower success rates per cycle.

- Limited efficacy in severe male factor infertility: In cases of severe male factor infertility, IVF may be more appropriate.

- Multiple birth risk: IUI increases the risk of multiple pregnancies, which may result in more complex pregnancies and deliveries.

Section 6

How to increase the Success rate of IUI Treatment

The success rates of IUI can vary depending on factors such as the woman's age, the cause of infertility, and the number of cycles attempted. On average, the success rate per cycle can range from 5% to 15%, with higher success rates for couples with specific fertility issues. Remember, this number can be higher or lower depending on various factors, such as:

- **Age:** Younger women generally have higher success rates with IUI compared to older women, as ovarian reserve and egg quality decline with age.They may require fewer cycles to achieve pregnancy compared to older women. Other than the reason for infertility, age is the most important factor in determining the success of IUI. Most healthcare providers will recommend IUI before turning 40 to increase your chance of becoming pregnant. As a person ages, they have fewer eggs and the quality of those eggs decreases. The pregnancy rate for IUI by age is:

- Age 20 to 30: 17.6%
  - Age 31 to 35: 13.3%
  - Age 36 to 38: 13.4%
  - Age 39 to 40: 10.6%
  - Over 40: 5.4%

- **Fertility diagnosis:** The underlying cause of infertility can impact the success of IUI. If the cause is treatable with IUI, the likelihood of success increases.

- **Sperm quality:** The quality of the sperm used in the IUI procedure, including sperm count and motility, can affect the chances of successful fertilization.

Factors that may influence the duration of the treatment

Several factors can impact the duration of an IUI treatment, such as:

- **Age of the woman:** Younger women typically respond better to fertility medications.

- **Cause of infertility:** The underlying cause of infertility can influence the success and duration of IUI treatment. If the cause is easily treatable, the treatment may be shorter.

- **Ovulation response:** The woman's response to ovulation-stimulating medications can vary. Some may require adjustments to medication dosages or additional monitoring, which can extend the treatment timeline.

- **The number of IUI Cycles attempted:** Success with IUI may require multiple cycles. If previous attempts are unsuccessful, the doctor may recommend further cycles.

How to minimize the risks during the procedure

To minimize the risks associated with IUI, it is essential to follow certain precautions:

- Expert Medical Guidance: Seek treatment from a qualified fertility specialist with experience in IUI procedures.

- Monitoring: Regular monitoring throughout the IUI treatment cycle helps identify any potential complications early.

- Hormonal Dosage: Precise adjustment of hormonal medication dosages helps reduce the risk of OHSS.

- Semen Analysis: Thorough evaluation of the sperm sample ensures the use of the healthiest and most motile sperm.

What to do if IUI is unsuccessful?

If an IUI cycle does not result in pregnancy, several options are available for consideration:

Reevaluating the treatment plan: The fertility specialist may review the treatment plan and make adjustments based on the individual's response to the previous cycle.

Considering additional cycles: Depending on the fertility diagnosis and other factors, the doctor may discuss the decision to attempt additional IUI cycles or consider alternative treatments, such as IVF.

Seeking support: Coping with an unsuccessful IUI cycle can be emotionally challenging.

Seeking support from a counselor or support group can provide valuable guidance during this time.

The Risks Factors of IUI after Treatment

While IUI is generally considered safe, there are some potential risks and complications:

- **Risk of multiple pregnancies:** IUI may result in multiple pregnancies (e.g., twins or triplets), which can carry higher risks for both the mother and the babies.

- **Ovarian Hyperstimulation Syndrome (OHSS):** In some cases, ovulation-stimulating medications can lead to OHSS, a condition where the ovaries become swollen and painful.

- **Infection**: There is a slight risk of infection during or after the procedure.

- **Spotting:** The procedure can cause a small amount of vaginal bleeding.

What are the common side effects experienced with IUI?

While IUI is generally a well-tolerated procedure, some women may experience mild side effects. Common side effects include:

- Mild Cramping: Some women may experience mild cramping during or after the IUI procedure. This discomfort is typically short-lived.
- Spotting or Light Bleeding: Light spotting or vaginal bleeding may occur after the procedure, but it should resolve quickly.
- Emotional changes: The hormonal changes and anticipation of the procedure can lead to emotional fluctuations, such as feeling anxious, excited, or even disappointed.

One must rest and hydrate after the procedure to ease the discomfort. Also, if they experience pain and discomfort, the doctor may prescribe over-the-counter pain relievers. Lastly, if the symptoms persist, they must consult the doctor.

Section 7

Recovery and Outlook

How effective is IUI in getting pregnant

IUI can be highly effective, especially when fertility drugs are used. The pregnancy rate for IUI when fertility drugs are used can be as high as 20%. The effectiveness of IUI is mostly dependent on the underlying cause of infertility and the age of the birth parent. The IUI fertility rate is about the same as a normal conception (around 20%), which means IUI helps bring people's chances up to a more typical success rate.

How long does it take to know you are pregnant after IUI?

You'll know if you're pregnant approximately two weeks after IUI. It takes about that long for human chorionic gonadotropin (hCG) to be detected in blood or urine. Your healthcare provider will let you know if you should return for a blood test to detect pregnancy or if you can use an at-home urine test.

How many cycles of IUI do you try before IVF?

Most healthcare providers recommend three cycles of IUI before pursuing another reproductive treatment, like IVF. If you're over the age of 40, some healthcare providers recommend just one cycle of IUI before moving on to IVF. This is because the success rates for IVF are higher for that age group and timely treatment is important.

In some cases, going straight to IVF treatment and skipping IUI may be better for you. This is the case if you have a condition like endometriosis, fallopian tube damage or advanced maternal age.

If you haven't gotten pregnant after three cycles of IUI, your healthcare provider will discuss the next steps with you.

Sex after IUI

Yes, you can have sex before and after IUI. You're increasing your chances of becoming pregnant by having sex the day of IUI or the day after.

When to Call the Doctor

If you're taking fertility medications for IUI, you should contact your healthcare provider if any of the following happens:

- Severe pelvic or abdominal pain.
- Nausea and vomiting.
- Shortness of breath.
- Sudden weight gain.
- Dizziness or lightheadedness.

If you're having difficulty conceiving, speak with your healthcare provider. Many people struggle with infertility, and there are options to help you. IUI may be one of those options. Your healthcare provider will work with you to determine the right fertility treatment to help you achieve a successful pregnancy.

FAQ on IUI (Intrauterine Insemination)

Can individuals with diabetes undergo IUI?

Yes. Individuals with diabetes can undergo IUI, but careful monitoring and management of blood sugar levels are essential to ensure a successful procedure and healthy pregnancy.

Can IUI be done if someone has kidney issues?

Yes. IUI can be considered for individuals with kidney issues, but close medical supervision is crucial to manage any potential complications and ensure a safe pregnancy.

Can weak bones influence IUI outcomes?

While bone health itself may not directly affect IUI outcomes, maintaining good overall health, including bone health, is important for a successful pregnancy. Adequate calcium and vitamin D intake can support both fertility and pregnancy.

How does liver health affect IUI success?

Liver health can indirectly impact IUI success by affecting overall well-being. Individuals with liver conditions should consult their healthcare provider before undergoing IUI to ensure optimal health for pregnancy.

Is IUI safe for individuals with heart conditions?

IUI can be safe for individuals with stable heart conditions, but a thorough evaluation by a cardiologist is recommended to assess the risks and ensure that the procedure can be performed safely without putting additional strain on the heart.

Is IUI safe for individuals with high cholesterol?

Yes. IUI is generally safe for individuals with high cholesterol. However, it's important to manage cholesterol levels through proper diet and medication to reduce any potential impact on fertility and pregnancy.